Table of Contents

Introduction

New research in mice suggests that keeping blood sugar under control using either the ketogenic diet or a diabetes drug could help treat certain cancers by boosting the efficacy of standard chemotherapy.The ketogenic diet consists of high fat foods, foods that contain an adequate amount of protein, and a very low amount of carbohydrates.Normally, the human body gets its main source of energy (sugar) from carbs.However, the ketogenic diet deprives the body of glucose, inducing a state of "ketosis." During ketosis, the body is forced to break down stored fat instead of sugar to produce an alternative source of energy. The ketogenic, or "keto," diet has been around for centuries. Traditionally, some have used it as a therapy for conditions such as diabetes and epilepsy. Newer studies have started to examine the therapeutic potential of the keto diet for other conditions, such as cancer, polycystic ovary syndrome, and Alzheimer's disease.

The keto diet is a very low-carb and higher-fat diet.It's similar in many ways to other low-carb diets. While you eat far fewer carbohydrates on a keto diet, you maintain moderate levels of protein intake and may increase your intake of fat. The reduction in carb intake puts your body in a metabolic state called ketosis, where fat, from your diet and from your body, is burned for energy.

What "Keto" Means

The "keto" in a ketogenic diet comes from the fact that it allows the body to produce small fuel molecules called "ketones." This is an alternative fuel source for the body, used when blood sugar (glucose) is in short supply. When you eat very few carbs or very few calories, the liver produces ketones from fat.These ketones then serve as a fuel source throughout the body, especially for the brain. The brain is a hungry organ that consumes lots of energy every day, and it can't run on fat directly. It can only run on glucose – or ketones. On a ketogenic diet, your entire body switches its fuel supply to run mostly on fat, burning fat 24-7. When insulin levels become very low, fat burning can increase dramatically.It becomes easier to access your fat stores to burn them off. This is great if you're trying to lose weight, but there can also be other, less obvious benefits, such as less hunger and a steady supply of energy (without the sugar peaks and valleys we can get from high carb meals). This may help keep you alert and focused. When the body produces ketones, it enters a metabolic state called ketosis. The fastest way to get there is by fasting – not eating anything – but nobody can consistently fast forever.A keto diet, on the other hand, also results in ketosis and can be eaten indefinitely.It has many of the benefits of fasting – including weight loss – without having to fast long-term.

There are controversies and myths about a keto diet, but for most people it appears to be very safe. However, three groups often require special consideration:

• People taking medication for diabetes, e.g. insulin

• People taking medication for high blood pressure

• If you breastfeeding

You should base the majority of your meals around these foods:

• Meat: Red meat, steak, ham, sausage, bacon, chicken and turkey.

• Fatty fish: Such as salmon, trout, tuna and mackerel.

• Eggs: Look for pastured or omega-3 whole eggs.

• Butter and cream: Look for grass-fed when possible.

• Cheese: Unprocessed cheese (cheddar, goat, cream, blue or mozzarella).

• Nuts and seeds: Almonds, walnuts, flax seeds, pumpkin seeds, chia seeds, etc.

• Healthy oils: Primarily extra virgin olive oil, coconut oil and avocado oil.

• Avocados: Whole avocados or freshly made guacamole.

• Low-carb veggies: Most green veggies, tomatoes, onions, peppers, etc.

• Condiments: You can use salt, pepper and various healthy herbs and spices.

It is best to base your diet mostly on whole, single-ingredient foods.

Foods To Avoid

Any food that is high in carbs should be limited. Here is a list of foods that need to be reduced or eliminated on a ketogenic diet:

• Sugary foods: Soda, fruit juice, smoothies, cake, ice cream, candy, etc.

• Grains or starches: Wheat-based products, rice, pasta, cereal, etc.

• Fruit: All fruit, except small portions of berries like strawberries.

• Beans or legumes: Peas, kidney beans, lentils, chickpeas, etc.

• Root vegetables and tubers: Potatoes, sweet potatoes, carrots, parsnips, etc.

• Low-fat or diet products: These are highly processed and often high in carbs.

• Some condiments or sauces: These often contain sugar and unhealthy fat.

• Unhealthy fats: Limit your intake of processed vegetable oils, mayonnaise, etc.

• Alcohol: Due to their carb content, many alcoholic beverages can throw you out of ketosis.

• Sugar-free diet foods: These are often high in sugar alcohols, which can affect ketone levels in some cases. These foods also tend to be highly processed.

Healthy Keto Snacks

In case you get hungry between meals, here are some healthy, keto-approved snacks:

• Fatty meat or fish

• Cheese

• A handful of nuts or seeds

• Cheese with olives

• 1–2 hard-boiled eggs

• 90% dark chocolate

• A low-carb milkshake with almond milk, cocoa powder and nut butter

• Full-fat yogurt mixed with nut butter and cocoa powder

• Strawberries and cream

• Celery with salsa and guacamole

• Smaller portions of leftover meals

Keto Meal Plan For 1 Week

To help get you started, here is a sample ketogenic diet meal plan for one week:

Monday

• Breakfast: Bacon, eggs and tomatoes.

• Lunch: Chicken salad with olive oil and feta cheese.

• Dinner: Salmon with asparagus cooked in butter.

Tuesday

• Breakfast: Egg, tomato, basil and goat cheese omelet.

• Lunch: Almond milk, peanut butter, cocoa powder and stevia milkshake.

• Dinner: Meatballs, cheddar cheese and vegetables.

Wednesday

• Breakfast: A ketogenic milkshake (try this or this).

• Lunch: Shrimp salad with olive oil and avocado.

• Dinner: Pork chops with Parmesan cheese, broccoli and salad.

Thursday

• Breakfast: Omelet with avocado, salsa, peppers, onion and spices.

• Lunch: A handful of nuts and celery sticks with guacamole and salsa.

• Dinner: Chicken stuffed with pesto and cream cheese, along with vegetables.

Friday

• Breakfast: Sugar-free yogurt with peanut butter, cocoa powder and stevia.

• Lunch: Beef stir-fry cooked in coconut oil with vegetables.

• Dinner: Bun-less burger with bacon, egg and cheese.

Saturday

• Breakfast: Ham and cheese omelet with vegetables.

• Lunch: Ham and cheese slices with nuts.

• Dinner: White fish, egg and spinach cooked in coconut oil.

Sunday

• Breakfast: Fried eggs with bacon and mushrooms.

• Lunch: Burger with salsa, cheese and guacamole.

• Dinner: Steak and eggs with a side salad.

Always try to rotate the vegetables and meat over the long term, as each type provides different nutrients and health benefits.

An Overview Of Ketosis

First, it's necessary to understand what ketosis is. Ketosis is a natural part of metabolism. It happens either when carbohydrate intake is very low (such as on a ketogenic diet), or when you haven't eaten for a long time. Both of these lead to reduced insulin levels, which causes a lot of fat to be released from your fat cells. When this happens, the liver gets flooded with fat, which turns a large part of it into ketones. During ketosis, many parts of your body are burning ketones for energy instead of carbs. This includes a large part of the brain. However, this doesn't happen instantly. It takes your body and brain some time to "adapt" to burning fat and ketones instead of carbs. During this adaptation phase, you may experience some temporary side effects. These are generally referred to as the "low-carb flu" or "keto flu."

How To Get Into Ketosis On A Keto Diet

Here are the seven most important things to increase your level of ketosis, ranked from most to least important:

• Restrict carbohydrates to 20 digestible grams per day or less – a strict low-carb or keto diet. Fiber does not have to be restricted; it might even be beneficial for ketosis.

• Eat enough fat to feel satisfied. A keto low-carb diet is normally a higher-fat diet, because fat supplies the energy that you are no longer getting from carbs. This is the big difference between a keto diet and starvation, which also results in ketosis. A keto diet is sustainable while starvation is not. If you feel as if you're starving, you're likely to feel tired and want to give up your diet. But a ketogenic diet should not result in hunger, making it sustainable and possibly making you feel great. So, eat enough protein foods and low-carb veggies, with enough added fat to feel satisfied. If you're hungry all the time, check that you are getting adequate amounts of protein at most meals and, if so, add more fat to your meals (like more butter, more olive oil, or some delicious sauces).

• Maintain a moderate protein intake. A keto diet is not meant to be a very high protein diet. We recommend 1.2 to 1.7 grams per kg of reference body weight per day. This means about 100 grams of protein per day if your lean body mass weight is around 70 kilos (155 pounds). Despite concerns that people on keto diets eat "too much" protein, this does not seem to be the case for most people. Because it is very filling, most people find it difficult to overeat protein. Although amino acids from protein foods can be converted to glucose, under experimental conditions, only a small percentage actually are. This may be related to individual factors, such as degree of insulin resistance. However, even people with type 2 diabetes usually do well with the adequate levels of protein, if their diets are also low carb. At the same time, inadequate protein intake over extended periods of time is a serious concern. It can result in loss of muscle and bone, especially as you age.

• Avoid snacking when not hungry. Eating more often than you need, just eating for fun, or eating because there's food around, reduces ketosis and slows down weight loss. Though using keto snacks may minimize the damage when you're hungry between meals, try to adjust your meals so that snacks become unnecessary.

• If necessary, add intermittent fasting. For example, skip breakfast and only eat during 8 hours of the day, fasting for 16 hours (i.e. 16:8 fasting). This is effective at boosting ketone levels, as well as accelerating weight loss and improving insulin resistance. It's also usually easy to do on keto.

• Add exercise. Adding any kind of physical activity while on low carb can increase ketone levels moderately. It can also help speed up weight loss and improve type 2 diabetes. Exercise is not necessary to get into ketosis, but it may be helpful.

• Sleep enough and minimize stress. Most people benefit from a minimum of seven hours of sleep per night on average. And try to keep stress under control. Sleep deprivation and stress hormones raise blood sugar levels, slowing ketosis and weight loss. Plus, they might make it harder to stick to a keto diet and resist temptations. So, while handling sleep and stress will not get you into ketosis on their own, they are still worth thinking about.

• Keto supplements are not required. Note what's not on the list above: you do not need expensive supplements, like exogenous ketones or MCT oil (medium-chain triglycerides). These supplements will likely not help you lose weight or reverse disease. At least there's no evidence for that.

How To Know You're In Ketosis

How do you know if you're in ketosis? It's possible to measure it by testing urine, blood or breath samples. But there are also telltale symptoms that require no testing:

• Dry mouth and increased thirst. Unless you drink enough water and get enough electrolytes like salt, you may feel a dry mouth. Try a cup of bouillon or two daily, plus as much water as you need. You may also feel a metallic taste in your mouth.

• Increased urination. A ketone body, acetoacetate, may end up in the urine. This makes it possible to test for ketosis using urine strips. It also – at least when starting out – can result in having to go to the bathroom more often. This may be the main cause of the increased thirst (above).

• Keto breath. This is due to a ketone body called acetone escaping via our breath. It can make a person's breath smell "fruity," or similar to nail polish remover. This smell can sometimes also come from sweat, when working out. It's often temporary. Learn more

Other, less specific but more positive signs include:

• Reduced hunger. Many people experience a marked reduction in hunger on a keto diet. In fact, many people feel great when they eat just once or twice a day, and may automatically end up doing a form of intermittent fasting.

This saves time and money, while also speeding up weight loss.

• Possibly increased energy. After a few days of feeling tired (the "keto flu") many people experience a clear increase in energy levels. This can also be experienced as clear thinking, a lack of "brain fog," or even a sense of euphoria.

Ketosis Safety And Side Effects

Some people think that ketosis is extremely dangerous. However, they might be confusing ketosis with ketoacidosis, which is completely different. While ketoacidosis is a serious condition caused by uncontrolled diabetes, ketosis is a natural metabolic state. In fact, ketosis and ketogenic diets have been studied extensively and shown to have major benefits for weight loss. Ketogenic diets have also been shown to have therapeutic effects in epilepsy, type 2 diabetes and several other chronic conditions. Ketosis is generally considered to be safe for most people. However, it may lead to a few side effects, especially in the beginning.

In the beginning of ketosis, you may experience a range of negative symptoms. They are often referred to as "low-carb flu" or "keto flu" because they resemble symptoms of the flu. These may include:

• Headache.

• Fatigue.

• Brain fog.

• Increased hunger.

• Poor sleep.

• Nausea.

• Decreased physical performance.

These issues may discourage people from continuing to follow a ketogenic diet, even before they start reaping all the benefits. However, the "low-carb flu" is usually over within a few days.

Bad Breath

One of the more common side effects of ketosis is bad breath, often described as fruity and slightly sweet. It's caused by acetone, a ketone that is a byproduct of fat metabolism. Blood acetone levels are elevated in ketosis, and your body gets rid of some of it via your breath. Occasionally, sweat and urine can also start to smell like acetone. Acetone has a distinctive smell — it's the chemical that gives nail polish remover its pungent odor. For most people, this unusual-smelling breath will go away within a few weeks.

Leg Muscles May Cramp

In ketosis, some people may experience leg cramps. Although they're usually a minor problem, they're never pleasant and can be painful. Leg cramps in ketosis are usually connected to dehydration and loss of mincrals. This is because ketosis causes a reduction in water weight. Glycogen, the storage form of glucose in muscles and liver, binds water. This gets flushed out when you reduce carb intake, and is one of the main reasons why people lose weight rapidly in the first week of a very low-carb diet. That being said, there are many other potential causes of muscle cramps.

Ketosis May Cause Digestive Problems

Dietary changes can sometimes lead to digestive issues. This is also true for ketogenic diets, and constipation is a common side effect in the beginning. This is most commonly due to not eating enough fiber and not drinking enough fluids. Some people may also get diarrhea, but it's less common. If you made drastic changes to your diet in order to get into ketosis, it's more likely that you'll experience digestive symptoms. Nevertheless, digestive issues are usually over within a few weeks.

Elevated Heart Rate

Some people also experience increased heart rate as a side effect of ketosis. This is also called heart palpitations or a racing heart, and can happen during the first few weeks of a ketogenic diet. Being dehydrated is a common cause, as well as low salt intake. Drinking a lot of coffee might also contribute to this. If the problem doesn't stop, you might need to increase your carb intake.

Other Side Effects of Ketosis

Other, less common side effects may include:

• Ketoacidosis: A few cases of ketoacidosis (a serious condition that occurs in uncontrolled diabetes) have been reported in breastfeeding women, likely triggered by a very low-carb diet. However, this is extremely rare.

• Kidney stones: Although uncommon, some epileptic children have developed kidney stones on a ketogenic diet.

• Raised cholesterol levels: Some people get increased total and low-density lipoprotein (LDL) cholesterol levels.

How to Minimize Potential Side Effects

Here's how to minimize the potential side effects of ketosis:

• Drink plenty of water: Make sure to drink at least 68 oz (2 liters) of water a day. A significant amount of water weight is lost in ketosis, especially in the beginning.

• Get enough salt: Sodium, a crucial electrolyte, gets excreted in large amounts when carb intake is reduced. Replenish your salt by adding it to foods or drinking broth.

• Increase mineral intake: Foods high in magnesium and potassium may help relieve leg cramps.

• Avoid intense exercise: Don't push yourself too hard while you're adapting to ketosis. Stick to moderate levels of exercise in the first week or two.

• Try a low-carb diet first: To ease the transition, it might help to reduce your carbs to a moderate amount before trying a ketogenic (very low-carb) diet.

• Eat fiber: A low-carb diet is not no-carb. Eat fiber-rich foods like nuts, seeds, berries and low-carb veggies.

Ketosis Is Healthy and Safe, but Is Not Suitable for Everyone

Being in ketosis has been shown to have powerful benefits for certain people, such as people with obesity or type 2 diabetes and children with epilepsy. Yet although ketosis is generally healthy and safe, you may experience some side effects. These include the "low-carb flu," leg cramps, bad breath and digestive issues. However, these effects are usually temporary and should go away within a few days or weeks. Diet and lifestyle changes can also help minimize these effects. Additionally, it should be noted that while getting into ketosis has obvious benefits for some people, it is definitely not for everyone. Some people feel great and experience incredible benefits on a ketogenic diet, while others feel and perform much better on a higher-carb diet.

Keto Flu

The keto flu is a collection of symptoms experienced by some people when they first start the keto diet. These symptoms, which can feel similar to the flu, are caused by the body adapting to a new diet consisting of very little carbohydrates. Reducing your carb intake forces your body to burn ketones for energy instead of glucose. Ketones are byproducts of fat breakdown and become the main fuel source when following a ketogenic diet. Normally, fat is reserved as a secondary fuel source to use when glucose is not available. This switch to burning fat for energy is called ketosis. It occurs during specific circumstances, including starvation and fasting. However, ketosis can also be reached by adopting a very low-carb diet. In a ketogenic diet, carbohydrates are typically reduced to under 50 grams per day. This drastic reduction can come as a shock to the body and may cause withdrawal-like symptoms, similar to those experienced when weaning off an addictive substance like caffeine.

Symptoms

Switching to a very low-carb diet is a major change, and your body may need time to adapt to this new way of eating. For some people, this transition period can be especially difficult. Signs of the keto flu may start popping up within the first few days of cutting back on carbs. Symptoms can range from mild to severe and vary from person to person. While some people may transition to a ketogenic diet without any side effects, others may experience one or more of the following symptoms:

• Nausea

• Vomiting

• Constipation

• Diarrhea

• Headache

• Irritability

• Weakness

• Muscle cramps

• Dizziness

• Poor concentration

• Stomach pain

• Muscle soreness

• Difficulty sleeping

• Sugar cravings

These symptoms are commonly reported by those who have just begun the ketogenic diet and can be distressing. Symptoms typically last about a week, though some people may experience them for a longer period of time. While these side effects may cause some dieters to throw in the towel, there are ways to reduce them.

How to Get Rid of the Keto Flu

The keto flu can make you feel miserable. Luckily, there are ways to reduce its flu-like symptoms and help your body get through the transition period more easily.

Stay Hydrated: Drinking enough water is necessary for optimal health and can also help reduce symptoms. A keto diet can cause you to rapidly shed water stores, increasing the risk of dehydration. This is because glycogen, the stored form of carbohydrates, binds to water in the body.

When dietary carbohydrates are reduced, glycogen levels plummet and water is excreted from the body. Staying hydrated can help with symptoms like fatigue and muscle cramping. Replacing fluids is especially important when you are experiencing keto-flu-associated diarrhea, which can cause additional fluid loss.

Avoid Strenuous Exercise: While exercise is important for staying healthy and keeping body weight in check, strenuous exercise should be avoided when experiencing keto-flu symptoms. Fatigue, muscle cramps and stomach discomfort are common in the first week of following a ketogenic diet, so it may be a good idea to give your body a rest. Activities like intense biking, running, weight lifting and strenuous workouts may have to be put on the back burner while your system adapts to new fuel sources. While these types of exercise should be avoided if you are experiencing the keto flu, light activities like walking, yoga or leisurely biking may improve symptoms.

Replace Electrolytes: Replacing dietary electrolytes may help reduce keto-flu symptoms. When following a ketogenic diet, levels of insulin, an important hormone that helps the body absorb glucose from the bloodstream, decrease. When insulin levels decrease, the kidneys release excess sodium from the body. What's more, the keto diet restricts many foods that are high in potassium, including fruits, beans and starchy vegetables. Getting adequate amounts of these important nutrients is an excellent way to power through the adaptation period of the diet. Salting food to taste and including potassium-rich, keto-friendly foods like green leafy vegetables and avocados are an excellent way to ensure you are maintaining a healthy balance of electrolytes. These foods are also high in magnesium, which may help reduce muscle cramps, sleep issues and headaches.

Get Adequate Sleep: Fatigue and irritability are common complaints of people who are adapting to a ketogenic diet. Lack of sleep causes levels of the stress hormone cortisol to rise in the body, which can negatively impact mood and make keto-flu symptoms worse. If you are having a difficult time falling or staying asleep, try one of the following tips:

• Reduce caffeine intake: Caffeine is a stimulant that may negatively impact sleep. If you drink caffeinated beverages, only do so in the morning so your sleep is not affected.

• Cut out ambient light: Shut off cell phones, computers and televisions in the bedroom to create a dark environment and promote restful sleep.

• Take a bath: Adding Epsom salt or lavender essential oil to your bath is a relaxing way to wind down and get ready for sleep.

• Get up early: Waking at the same time every day and avoiding oversleeping may help normalize your sleep patterns and improve sleep quality over time.

Make Sure You Are Eating Enough Fat (and Carbs): Transitioning to a very low-carb diet can cause you to crave foods that are restricted on the ketogenic diet, such as cookies, bread, pasta and bagels. However, eating enough fat, the primary fuel source on the ketogenic diet, will help reduce cravings and keep you feeling satisfied. In fact, research shows that low-carb diets help reduce cravings for sweets and high-carb foods. Those having a difficult time adapting to the ketogenic diet may have to eliminate carbohydrates gradually, rather than all at once. Slowly cutting back on carbs, while increasing fat and protein in your diet, may help make the transition smoother and decrease keto-flu symptoms.

How People Get the Keto Flu

People adapt to ketogenic diets differently. While some may experience weeks of keto-flu symptoms, others may adjust to the new diet with no adverse side effects. The symptoms people experience is tied to how their bodies adjust to a new fuel source. Usually, carbs provide the body with energy in the form of glucose. When carbs are substantially reduced, the body burns ketones from fat instead of glucose. Those who typically consume lots of carbs, especially refined carbs like pasta, sugary cereal and soda, may have a more difficult time when beginning the ketogenic diet. Thus, the transition to a high-fat, very low-carb diet may be a struggle for some, while others are able to switch between fuel sources easily with little to no keto-flu symptoms. The reason some people adapt to ketogenic diets easier than others is unknown, but genetics, electrolyte loss, dehydration and carbohydrate withdrawal are believed to be the driving forces behind the keto flu.

Luckily, the uncomfortable symptoms of the keto flu only last about a week for most people. However, some people may have a more difficult time adapting to this high-fat, low-carb diet. For these individuals, symptoms may last several weeks. Fortunately, these symptoms will gradually decrease as your body gets used to converting ketones into energy. While keto-flu symptoms are commonly reported by those shifting to a ketogenic diet, if you are feeling particularly unwell and experiencing symptoms like prolonged diarrhea, fever or vomiting, it's best to contact your doctor to rule out other causes.

Supplements For Keto Diets

Some supplements, such as medium chain triglyceride (MCT) oil and omega-3 fatty acids, can increase the effectiveness of the keto diet and help people achieve the intended ratio of fat in their diet. As the keto diet limits or eliminates many different foods, people who follow this diet can also use supplements to fill in any nutritional gaps. Magnesium, electrolytes, and fiber may be especially important. Adjusting to extreme carbohydrate restriction can cause uncomfortable side effects because the body takes time to get used to making ketones and using this new source of energy. The body usually burns carbohydrates for energy, but when a person eats few to no carbs on the keto diet, the body must get its energy from other sources. So, the body burns fat and turns it into ketones, which it can then use for energy. This process is called ketosis. Certain supplements, such as electrolytes, digestive enzymes, and L-theanine, may help minimize these symptoms. The following supplements may be helpful for people on a keto diet:

Medium chain triglyceride oil

Medium chain triglyceride oil, or MCT oil, is a type of fatty acid that occurs in coconut oil. The liver metabolizes these fats, transforming them into a source of fuel. A 2018 study found a "clear ketogenic effect" when people took supplemental MCTs. MCTs may also help a person lose more weight, according to some research. MCTs are not in many other foods, so taking a supplement can allow a person to get the potential benefits of these fats. MCT oil is liquid at room temperature. People can mix it into foods or smoothies, or they can take it alone. A standard dose is 1 teaspoon. People should try this to start because a higher initial dose, such as 1 tablespoon or more, may induce diarrhea.

Magnesium

Magnesium is a mineral and electrolyte that is abundant in the body. The body needs magnesium for many different processes, including food metabolism, transmission of nerve signals, balance of fluids, maintenance of bone and muscle health, and more. Although a few keto friendly foods, such as nuts and spinach, are high in magnesium, the diet is low in other magnesium rich foods, including whole grains, fruit, beans, and dairy products. If a person is not getting adequate magnesium from foods while following the keto diet, they may need a supplement. A supplement may also be beneficial for those experiencing constipation. Some evidence suggests that many people are at a high risk of magnesium deficiency due to chronic diseases, medications, and decreases in food crop magnesium levels. Magnesium supplements are available in different forms. The Office of Dietary Supplements (ODS) state that the body may absorb some types — including magnesium aspartate, citrate, lactate, glycinate, and chloride forms — more readily than others. However, a doctor may recommend a specific form of magnesium to meet a person's needs. High doses of magnesium can cause diarrhea. Therefore, a person should start with the lowest dose on the package, which may be 100–200 milligrams (mg) per day. If no diarrhea occurs, a person may gradually increase the dose, although they should not take more than 400 mg per day unless a doctor advises a higher dose.

Electrolytes

As the body adjusts to a keto diet, the kidneys may excrete more water. This increased excretion can cause the body to lose vital electrolytes, which include not only magnesium but also potassium, chloride, phosphorus, and sodium. Taking an electrolyte supplement can help rebalance the levels of these minerals. Electrolyte supplements vary in their mineral content, so it is important for a person to read labels to be sure that they are not getting too much of these minerals. Most contain a combination of calcium, potassium, and magnesium. A keto friendly supplement should contain no sugar or sweeteners. Alternatively, a person may wish to try adopting the following practices to get the three main electrolytes:

• taking a magnesium supplement daily

• adding some extra salt to the diet or consuming beef or chicken broth daily

• eating potassium rich, keto friendly foods, such as avocado or cooked spinach, every day

Fiber

Fiber is the indigestible part of plant foods, and it is important for keeping the digestive system healthy. Without enough fiber, a person may become constipated. People should get 25–31 grams of fiber per day, depending on their age and sex. Many keto friendly foods, including nuts, seeds, avocado, and leafy greens, contain fiber. However, if a person focuses on meat, seafood, eggs, and dairy, they may not get enough fiber on the keto diet. Fiber supplements can be helpful if people find that they become constipated while following the keto diet. They should look for a keto friendly formula that does not contain sugar. It is also important to drink plenty of water, which helps keep digestion running smoothly. Taking fiber supplements without adequate water intake could make constipation worse.

Omega-3 fatty acids

Omega-3 fats are a type of polyunsaturated fatty acid (PUFA). Omega-3s are present in high amounts in some fatty fish and eggs, and they also occur in plant form in some nuts and seeds. Studies show that consuming enough omega-3s can have health benefits, including helping prevent weight gain. The ODS state that many people could benefit from a higher intake of omega-3s. The other type of PUFA, omega-6, occurs in many conventionally raised, grain-fed meats.Omega-6s are also in some vegetable oils, including corn and cottonseed oil. One study found that among people following a ketogenic Mediterranean diet, those who ate more omega-3s experienced positive effects on their insulin, triglyceride, and inflammation levels. Omega-3 levels may be higher in meats that come from grass-fed or pasture raised animals, as well as in eggs from pasture raised or vegetarian-fed hens.If a person on the keto diet does not eat grass-fed meats or seafood, they may want to consider an omega-3 supplement. Omega-3 supplements vary in their dosage and origin.Some come from fish oil, krill oil, algae, flaxseed, or other natural omega-3 sources.A person should follow the dosage directions on the product. People who take medications that affect blood clotting, such as blood thinners, should ask a doctor before using omega-3 supplements.People who are allergic to fish or shellfish should avoid supplements that contain fish oil, krill oil, or other fish-based ingredients.

Digestive enzymes

The gut uses enzymes to break down different parts of foods during digestion. If a person who is switching to a keto diet ate a large number of carbs previously, they might find that they have trouble with the change. Symptoms such as bloating, nausea, fatigue, and constipation are common because of the high amount of fats that a keto diet requires. Digestive enzymes could help alleviate some of these symptoms. Many of these supplements contain several different types of enzyme, but it is important to choose one that contains lipase, which is the enzyme that breaks down fat. Supplements that contain proteases and peptidases are also a good choice, as these break down protein. In most cases, a person will take their digestive enzymes with a high fat meal or a few minutes before eating. They should always follow the dosage directions on the product and look for those that are keto friendly.

L-theanine

L-theanine is an amino acid that is difficult to obtain from foods. The only known good source of l-theanine is green or black tea, but the amounts may vary depending on the type of tea and how a person brews it. Studies show that taking this supplement may help improve sleep quality, decrease anxiety, and improve mental cognition. As a result, it could be an excellent option if a person experiences mental fog or trouble concentrating as they transition to the keto diet. L-theanine supplements are available in pill or powder form. There is no recommended dosage, but many products suggest 100–400 mg daily. Alternatively, people may choose to drink unsweetened tea, particularly green tea, which contains natural L-theanine.

Benefit Of Keto Diet

Supports weight loss

The ketogenic diet may help promote weight loss in several ways, including boosting metabolism and reducing appetite. Ketogenic diets consist of foods that fill a person up and may reduce hunger-stimulating hormones. For these reasons, following a keto diet may reduce appetite and promote weight loss. In a 2013 meta-analysis of 13 different randomized controlled trials, researchers found that people following ketogenic diets lost 2 pounds (lbs.) more than those following low fat diets over 1 year. Similarly, another review of 11 studies demonstrated that people following a ketogenic diet lost 5 lbs. more than those following low-fat diets after 6 months.

Improves acne

Acne has several different causes and may have links to diet and blood sugar in some people. Eating a diet high in processed and refined carbohydrates may alter the balance of gut bacteria and cause blood sugar to rise and fall significantly, both of which can adversely affect skin health. According to a 2012 study, by decreasing carb intake, a ketogenic diet could reduce acne symptoms in some people.

May reduce risk of certain cancers

Researchers have examined the effects of the ketogenic diet in helping prevent or even treat certain cancers. One study found that the ketogenic diet may be a safe and suitable complementary treatment to use alongside chemotherapy and radiation therapy in people with certain cancers. This is because it would cause more oxidative stress in cancer cells than in normal cells, causing them to die. A more recent study from 2018 suggests that because the ketogenic diet reduces blood sugar, it could also lower the risk of insulin complications. Insulin is a hormone that controls blood sugar that may have links to some cancers. Although some research indicates that the ketogenic diet may have some benefit in cancer treatment, studies in this area are limited. Researchers need to carry out more studies to fully understand the potential benefits of the ketogenic diet in cancer prevention and treatment.

May improve heart health

When a person follows the ketogenic diet, it is important that they choose healthful foods. Some evidence shows that eating healthful fats, such as avocados instead of less healthful fats, such as pork rinds, can help improve heart health by reducing cholesterol. A 2017 review of studies of animals and humans on a keto diet showed that some people experienced a significant drop in levels of total cholesterol, low-density lipoprotein (LDL), or bad cholesterol, and triglycerides, and an increase in high-density lipoprotein (HDL), or "good" cholesterol. High levels of cholesterol can increase the risk of cardiovascular disease. A keto diet's reducing effect on cholesterol may, therefore, reduce a person's risk of heart complications. However, the review concluded that the positive effects of the diet on heart health depend on diet quality. Therefore, it's important to eat healthful, nutritionally balanced food while following the keto diet.

May protect brain function

Some studies, such as this 2019 review, suggest the ketones that generate during the keto diet provide neuroprotective benefits, which means they can strengthen and protect the brain and nerve cells. For this reason, a keto diet may help a person prevent or manage conditions such as Alzheimer's disease. However, more research is necessary into a keto diet's effects on the brain.

Potentially reduces seizures

The ratio of fat, protein, and carbs in a keto diet alters the way the body uses energy, resulting in ketosis. Ketosis is a metabolic process during which the body uses ketone bodies for fuel. The Epilepsy Foundation suggest that

ketosis can reduce seizures in people with epilepsy —
especially those who have not responded to other treatment
methods. More research is necessary on how effective this
is, though it seems to have the most effect on children who
have focal seizures. A 2019 review supports the hypothesis
that a keto diet can support people with epilepsy. The
ketogenic diet may reduce epilepsy symptoms by several
different mechanisms.

Improves PCOS symptoms

Polycystic ovary syndrome (PCOS) is a hormonal disorder
that can lead to excess male hormones, ovulatory
dysfunction, and polycystic ovaries. A high-carbohydrate
diet can cause adverse effects in people with PCOS, such as
skin problems and weight gain. There are not many clinical
studies on the ketogenic diet and PCOS. One pilot study
from 2005 examined five women over 24 weeks. The
researchers found that a ketogenic diet improved several
markers of PCOS, including:

• weight loss

• hormone balance

• ratios of luteinizing hormone (LH) and follicle-stimulating hormone (FSH)

• levels of fasting insulin

A different review of studies from 2019 found that a keto diet had beneficial effects for people with hormonal disorders, including PCOS and type 2 diabetes. However, they did also caution that the studies were too diverse to recommend a keto diet as a general treatment for PCOS.

Cancer

Cancer causes cells to divide uncontrollably. This can result in tumors, damage to the immune system, and other impairment that can be fatal. In the United States, an estimated 15.5 million people with a history of cancer were living as of January 1, 2016, according to a 2018 report from the American Cancer Society. Cancer is a broad term. It describes the disease that results when cellular changes cause the uncontrolled growth and division of cells. Some types of cancer cause rapid cell growth, while others cause cells to grow and divide at a slower rate. Certain forms of cancer result in visible growths called tumors, while others, such as leukemia, do not. Most of the body's cells have specific functions and fixed lifespans. While it may sound like a bad thing, cell death is part of a natural and beneficial phenomenon called apoptosis. A cell receives instructions to die so that the body can replace it with a newer cell that functions better. Cancerous cells lack the components that instruct them to stop dividing and to die. As a result, they build up in the body, using oxygen and nutrients that would usually nourish other cells. Cancerous cells can form tumors, impair the immune system and cause other changes that prevent the body from functioning regularly. Cancerous cells may appear in one area, then spread via the lymph nodes. These are clusters of immune cells located throughout the body.

Types Of Cancer

The most common type of cancer in the U.S. is breast cancer, followed by lung and prostate cancers, according to the National Cancer Institute, which excluded nonmelanoma skin cancers from these findings. Each year, more than 40,000 people in the country receive a diagnosis of one of the following types of cancer:

• bladder

- colon and rectal

- endometrial

- kidney

- leukemia

- liver

- melanoma

- non-Hodgkin's lymphoma

- pancreatic

- thyroid

Other forms are less common. According to the National Cancer Institute, there are over 100 types of cancer.

Cancer development and cell division

Doctors classify cancer by:

- its location in the body

- the tissues that it forms in

For example, sarcomas develop in bones or soft tissues, while carcinomas form in cells that cover internal or external surfaces in the body. Basal cell carcinomas develop in the skin, while adenocarcinomas can form in the breast. When cancerous cells spread to other parts of the body, the medical term for this is metastasis. A person can also have more than one type of cancer at a time.

Risk Factors And Causes Of Cancer

Anything that may cause a normal body cell to develop abnormally potentially can cause cancer. Many things can cause cell abnormalities and have been linked to cancer development. Some cancer causes remain unknown while other cancers have environmental or lifestyle triggers or may develop from more than one known cause. Some may be developmentally influenced by a person's genetic makeup. Many patients develop cancer due to a combination of these factors. Although it is often difficult or impossible to determine the initiating event(s) that cause a cancer to develop in a specific person, research has provided clinicians with a number of likely causes that alone or in concert with other causes, are the likely candidates for initiating cancer. The following is a listing of major causes and is not all-inclusive as specific causes are routinely added as research advances:

• Chemical or toxic compound exposures: Benzene, asbestos, nickel, cadmium, vinyl chloride, benzidine, N-nitrosamines, tobacco or cigarette smoke (contains at least 66 known potential carcinogenic chemicals and toxins), asbestos, and aflatoxin

• Ionizing radiation: Uranium, radon, ultraviolet rays from sunlight, radiation from alpha, beta, gamma, and X-ray-emitting sources

• Pathogens: Human papillomavirus (HPV), EBV or Epstein-Barr virus, hepatitis viruses B and C, Kaposi's sarcoma-associated herpes virus (KSHV), Merkel cell polyomavirus, Schistosoma spp., and Helicobacter pylori; other bacteria are being researched as possible agents.

• Genetics: A number of specific cancers have been linked to human genes and are as follows: breast, ovarian, colorectal, prostate, skin and melanoma; the specific genes and other details are beyond the scope of this general article so the reader is referred to the National Cancer Institute for more details about genetics and cancer.

It is important to point out that most everyone has risk factors for cancer and is exposed to cancer-causing substances (for example, sunlight, secondary cigarette smoke, and X-rays) during their lifetime, but many individuals do not develop cancer. In addition, many people have the genes that are linked to cancer but do not develop it. Why? Although researchers may not be able give a satisfactory answer for every individual, it is clear that the higher the amount or level of cancer-causing materials a person is exposed to, the higher the chance the person will develop cancer. In addition, the people with genetic links to cancer may not develop it for similar reasons (lack of enough stimulus to make the genes function). In addition, some people may have a heightened immune response that controls or eliminates cells that are or potentially may become cancer cells. There is evidence that even certain dietary lifestyles may play a significant role in conjunction with the immune system to allow or prevent cancer cell survival. For these reasons, it is difficult to assign a specific cause of cancer to many individuals.

Recently, other risk factors have been added to the list of items that may increase cancer risk. Specifically, red meat (such as beef, lamb, and pork) was classified by the International Agency for Research on Cancer as a high-risk agent for potentially causing cancers; in addition, processed meats (salted, smoked, preserved, and/or cured meats) were placed on the carcinogenic list. Individuals that eat a lot of barbecued meat may also increase risk due to compounds formed at high temperatures. Other less defined situations that may increase the risk of certain cancers include obesity, lack of exercise, chronic inflammation, and hormones, especially those hormones used for replacement therapy. Other items such as cell phones have been heavily studied. In 2011, the World Health Organization classified cell phone low energy radiation as "possibly carcinogenic," but this is a very low risk level that puts cell phones at the same risk as caffeine and pickled vegetables.

Proving that a substance does not cause or is not related to increased cancer risk is difficult. For example, antiperspirants are considered to possibly be related to breast cancer by some investigators and not by others. The official stance by the NCI is "additional research is needed to investigate this relationship and other factors that may be involved." This unsatisfying conclusion is presented because the data collected so far is contradictory. Other claims that are similar require intense and expensive research that may never be done. Reasonable advice might be to avoid large amounts of any compounds even remotely linked to cancer, although it may be difficult to do in complex, technologically advanced modern societies.

Cancer Symptoms And Sign

Cancer often has no specific symptoms, so it is important that people limit their risk factors and undergo appropriate cancer screening. Most cancer screening is specific to certain age groups and your primary care doctor will know what screening to perform depending on your age. People with risk factors for cancer (for example, smokers, heavy alcohol use, high sun exposure, genetics) should be acutely aware of potential cancer symptoms and be evaluated by a physician if any develop. The best way to fight cancers is by prevention (eliminating or decreasing risk factors) and early detection. Cancer treatment advances every year and combined with early detection has made many cancers treatable. Consequently, individuals need to know which symptoms might point to cancer. People should not ignore a warning symptom that might lead to early diagnosis and possibly to a cure. Cancer gives most people no symptoms or signs that exclusively indicate the disease.

Unfortunately, every complaint or symptom of cancer can be explained by a harmless condition as well. Some cancers occur more frequently in certain age groups. If certain symptoms occur or persist, however, a doctor should be seen for further evaluation. Some common symptoms that may occur with cancer are as follows:

• Persistent cough or blood-tinged saliva: These symptoms usually represent simple infections such as bronchitis or sinusitis. They could be symptoms of lung cancer or head and neck cancer. Anyone with a nagging cough that lasts more than a month or with blood in the mucus that is coughed up should see a doctor.

• A change in bowel habits: Most changes in bowel habits are related to your diet and fluid intake. Doctors sometimes see pencil-thin stools with colon cancer. Occasionally, cancer exhibits continuous diarrhea. Some people with cancer feel as if they need to have a bowel movement and still feel that way after they have had a bowel movement. If any of these abnormal bowel complaints last more than a few days, they require evaluation. Any significant change in bowel habits that cannot be easily explained by dietary changes could be cancer-related and needs to be evaluated.

• Blood in the stool: A doctor always should investigate blood in your stool. Hemorrhoids frequently cause rectal bleeding, but because hemorrhoids are so common, they may exist with cancer. Therefore, even when you have hemorrhoids, you should have a doctor examine your entire intestinal tract when you have blood in your bowel movements. With some individuals, X-ray studies may be enough to clarify a diagnosis. Colonoscopy is usually recommended. Routine colonoscopy, even without symptoms, is recommended once you are 50 years old. Sometimes when the source of bleeding is entirely clear (for example, recurrent ulcers), these studies may not be needed.

• Unexplained anemia (low blood count): Anemia is a condition in which people have fewer than the expected number of red blood cells in their blood. Anemia should always be investigated. There are many kinds of anemia, but blood loss almost always causes iron deficiency anemia. Unless there is an obvious source of ongoing blood loss, this anemia needs to be explained. Many cancers can cause anemia, but bowel cancers most commonly cause iron deficiency anemia. Evaluation should include endoscopy or X-ray studies of your upper and lower intestinal tracts.

• Breast lump or breast discharge: Most breast lumps are noncancerous tumors such as fibroadenomas or cysts. But all breast lumps need to be thoroughly investigated for the possibility of breast cancer. A negative mammogram result is not usually sufficient to evaluate a breast lump. Your doctor needs to determine the appropriate X-ray study which might include an MRI or an ultrasound of the breast. Generally, diagnosis requires a needle aspiration or biopsy (a small tissue sample). Discharge from a breast is common, but some forms of discharge may be signs of cancer. If discharge is bloody or from only one nipple, further evaluation is recommended. Women are advised to conduct monthly breast self-examinations.

• Lumps in the testicles: Most men (90%) with cancer of the testicle have a painless or uncomfortable lump on a testicle. Some men have an enlarged testicle. Other conditions, such as infections and swollen veins, can also cause changes in your testicles, but any lump should be evaluated. Men are advised to conduct monthly testicular self-examinations.

• A change in urination: Urinary symptoms can include frequent urination, small amounts of urine, and slow urine flow or a general change in bladder function. These symptoms can be caused by urinary infections (usually in women) or, in men, by an enlarged prostate gland. Most men will suffer from harmless prostate enlargement as they age and will often have these urinary symptoms. These symptoms may also signal prostate cancer. Men experiencing urinary symptoms need further investigation, possibly including blood tests and a digital rectal exam. The PSA blood test, its indications, and interpretation of results should be discussed with your health care provider. If cancer is suspected, a biopsy of the prostate may be needed. Cancer of the bladder and pelvic tumors can also cause irritation of the bladder and urinary frequency.

Diagnosing Cancer

Often, a diagnosis begins when a person visits a doctor about an unusual symptom. The doctor will talk with the person about his or her medical history and symptoms. Then the doctor will do various tests to find out the cause of these symptoms. But many people with cancer have no symptoms. For these people, cancer is diagnosed during a medical test for another issue or condition. Sometimes a doctor finds cancer after a screening test in an otherwise healthy person. Examples of screening tests include colonoscopy, mammography, and a Pap test. A person may need more tests to confirm or disprove the result of the screening test. For most cancers, a biopsy is the only way to make a definite diagnosis. A biopsy is the removal of a small amount of tissue for further study. Learn more about making a diagnosis after a biopsy.

Treatments Of Cancer

Innovative research has fueled the development of new medications and treatment technologies. Doctors usually prescribe treatments based on the type of cancer, its stage at diagnosis, and the person's overall health. Below are examples of approaches to cancer treatment:

• Chemotherapy aims to kill cancerous cells with medications that target rapidly dividing cells. The drugs can also help shrink tumors, but the side effects can be severe.

• Hormone therapy involves taking medications that change how certain hormones work or interfere with the body's ability to produce them. When hormones play a significant role, as with prostate and breast cancers, this is a common approach.

• Immunotherapy uses medications and other treatments to boost the immune system and encourage it to fight cancerous cells. Two examples of these treatments are checkpoint inhibitors and adoptive cell transfer.

• Precision medicine, or personalized medicine, is a newer, developing approach. It involves using genetic testing to determine the best treatments for a person's particular presentation of cancer. Researchers have yet to show that it can effectively treat all types of cancer, however.

• Radiation therapy uses high-dose radiation to kill cancerous cells. Also, a doctor may recommend using radiation to shrink a tumor before surgery or reduce tumor-related symptoms.

• Stem cell transplant can be especially beneficial for people with blood-related cancers, such as leukemia or lymphoma. It involves removing cells, such as red or white blood cells, that chemotherapy or radiation has destroyed.

Lab technicians then strengthen the cells and put them back into the body.

• Surgery is often a part of a treatment plan when a person has a cancerous tumor. Also, a surgeon may remove lymph nodes to reduce or prevent the disease's spread.

• Targeted therapies perform functions within cancerous cells to prevent them from multiplying. They can also boost the immune system. Two examples of these therapies are small-molecule drugs and monoclonal antibodies.

Doctors will often employ more than one type of treatment to maximize effectiveness.

Tips For Cancer Prevention

While your diet is central to preventing cancer, other healthy habits can further lower your risk:

• Be as lean as possible without becoming underweight. Weight gain, overweight and obesity increases the risk of a number of cancers, including bowel, breast, prostate, pancreatic, endometrial, kidney, gallbladder, esophageal, and ovarian cancers.

• Be physically active for at least 30 minutes every day. Physical activity decreases the risk of colon, endometrial, and postmenopausal breast cancer. Three 10-minute sessions work just as well, but the key is to find an activity you enjoy and make it a part of your daily life.

• Limit alcoholic drinks. Limit consumption to no more than two drinks a day for men and one a day for women.

• Where possible, aim to meet nutritional needs through diet alone, instead of trying to use supplements to protect against cancer.

• It is best for mothers to breastfeed exclusively for up to 6 months and then add other liquids and foods. Babies who are breastfed are less likely to be overweight as children or adults.

• After treatment, cancer survivors should follow the recommendations for cancer prevention. Follow the recommendations for diet, healthy weight, and physical activity from your doctor or trained professional.

Keto Diet And Cancer

Keto Diet May Help Fight Certain Cancer Tumors

• Maintaining blood sugar levels can be helpful for your overall health.

• Early research also points to the benefits of keeping blood sugar levels low to help fight cancer.

• Past research has found that certain tumors may rely on high glucose levels.

Keeping blood sugar levels even throughout the day may help you avoid afternoon energy crashes. It might also ward off or help you manage diabetes. Now, early research published in the journal Cell Reports suggests that restricting your blood sugar might also help combat certain cancerous tumor growths. Researchers from the University of Texas at Dallas restricted blood sugar levels in mice by feeding them a ketogenic diet — one that's high in fat, moderate in protein, and low in carbs — and by giving them a diabetes drug that prevents the kidneys from reabsorbing glucose in the blood. The combination of the diet and diabetes drug didn't shrink the lung and esophageal cancers in the mice, but it did keep them from progressing. "Both the ketogenic diet and the pharmacological restriction of blood glucose by themselves inhibited the further growth of squamous cell carcinoma tumors in mice with lung cancer," Jung-Whan "Jay" Kim, PhD, corresponding author of the study and an assistant professor of biological sciences at UT Dallas, said in a press release. Both elements actually showed promise independent of one another, too. "The key finding of our new study in mice is that a ketogenic diet alone does have some tumor-growth inhibitory effect in squamous cell cancer," Kim said.

"When we combined this with the diabetes drug and chemotherapy, it was even more effective." However, Kim and his colleagues report that the keto diet and drug combination had no effect on non-squamous cell cancers. The research is in the extremely early stages. It's unclear if these results could be replicated in humans. But it joins a growing body of evidence finding that certain diets, including the keto diet, may act as a complementary therapy for some people undergoing cancer treatment.

A Secondary Finding Targets Sugar

This finding in particular suggests certain tumors might be susceptible to glucose restriction. It helps confirm earlier research by Kim and colleagues. Their 2017 study indicated that a certain type of cancer called squamous cell carcinoma (SCC) was particularly reliant on glucose to sustain itself and survive. As part of their research, Kim and investigators also took blood samples from 192 people who had SCC of the lung or esophagus, plus blood samples from 120 people with lung adenocarcinoma, another type of cancer. They measured the blood glucose levels in the samples and divided them by whether they were above or below 120 mg/dL, a common clinical measure of diabetes in blood sugar."Surprisingly, we found a robust correlation between higher blood-glucose concentration and worse survival among patients with squamous cell carcinoma," Kim said."We found no such correlation among the lung adenocarcinoma patients.This is an important observation that further implicates the potential efficacy of glucose restriction in attenuating squamous-cell cancer growth," he said.In other words, people who had SCC and a high blood glucose level had worse survival rates compared to people who had other types of cancer. This secondary finding indicates that blood glucose levels may also have an impact on the progression of cancer. Managing blood glucose levels during treatment may be an effective way to enhance conventional methods of cancer treatment. "Manipulating host glucose levels would be a new strategy that is different from just trying to kill cancer cells directly," Kim said. "I believe this is part of a paradigm shift from targeting cancer cells themselves. Immunotherapy is a good example of this, where the human immune system is activated to go after cancer cells."

The Keto Diet's Potential As Cancer Treatment

Cancer treatment and care have seen a shift in recent years. While conventional treatments like surgery, chemotherapy, and radiation are still the primary means for eliminating cancerous tumors, researchers are seeking out complementary methods that may help stop the growth of cells, or even help defeat them. These methods aren't thought of as a way to replace traditional therapies like radiation. Instead, they'd be an additional aid in the fight against cancer. In fact, one 2014 study already identified the keto diet "as an adjuvant therapy to conventional radiation and chemotherapies." In addition to helping regulate blood sugar levels, a keto diet could selectively induce metabolic oxidative stress in cancer cells. This could help make the cells more sensitive to treatments like chemotherapy and radiation. "Ketogenic diets are known to interfere with tumor growth in more ways than one," said Dr. William Li, author of "Eat to Beat Disease: The New Science of How Your Body Can Heal Itself.""Reducing glucose takes away a fuel source for cancer cells. Unlike healthy cells, abnormal cancer cells have difficulty adapting metabolically to a low glucose situation, compromising their ability to survive ."Li further explained, "But a ketogenic diet also triggers a chain reaction of at least three other cancer-fighting mechanisms. Less glucose means cells produce less IGF-1, a protein growth signal for cancer. Ketogenic diets also lower the tumor's ability to produce another growth signal called VEGF.

Tumors use this signal to grow a private blood supply. By cutting off the tumor blood supply, an effect called anti-angiogenesis, cancer cells become starved and can't grow." But the ketogenic diet shouldn't be considered standard care, says Quintin Pan, PhD, deputy scientific director at University Hospitals Seidman Cancer Center.It's too early to know if the benefits outweigh possible risks. "The anticancer benefits of a keto diet for cancer patients remain an open question and need to be addressed in a controlled clinical trial," Pan told Healthline. Pan also points out that the keto diet specifically is notoriously difficult to maintain. People undergoing cancer treatment should always talk with their doctor before trying a new strict diet and discuss potential issues that may arise for them. Many people receiving chemotherapy are nauseous; they may not be able to stick with a very strict diet. "Strict adherence to a keto diet is challenging, especially for cancer patients. And also, keto diets may lead to potential health risks," Pan said. "It is important for cancer patients to have a conversation with their clinician team, doctor, and dietitian before starting on a keto diet. " While there still needs to be more research, some experts are advising certain patients to see if the keto diet is right for them. Elena Villanueva, DC, a functional holistic medicine expert and founder of Modern Holistic Health, says some treatment facilities are beginning to use the diet because of anecdotal reports and preliminary data that show promising signs. "For those battling with cancer and for those who are in remission, the adaptation of a healthy ketogenic diet is showing many benefits," she said. "Several oncology centers around the country have implemented ketogenic diets combined with standard cancer treatments because of the anticancer effects from eliminating sugars from the diet."

Recipes

Sheet Pan Eggs With Veggies And Parmesan

• Servings: 6

• Prep Time: 5 minutes

• Cook Time: 15 minutes

Ingredients:

• 12 large eggs, whisked

• Salt and pepper

• 1 small red pepper, diced

• 1 small yellow onion, chopped

• 1 cup diced mushrooms

• 1 cup diced zucchini

• 1 cup freshly grated parmesan cheese

Instructions:

• Preheat the oven to 350°F and grease a rimmed baking sheet with cooking spray.

• Whisk the eggs in a bowl with salt and pepper until frothy.

• Stir in the peppers, onions, mushrooms, and zucchini until well combined.

• Pour the mixture in the baking sheet and spread into an even layer.

• Sprinkle with parmesan and bake for 12 to 15 minutes until the egg is set.

• Let cool slightly, then cut into squares to serve.

Nutrition Info: 215 calories, 14g fat, 18.5g protein, 5g carbs, 1g fiber, 4g net carbs

Bacon Cheeseburger Soup

• Servings: 4

• Prep Time: 10 minutes

• Cook Time: 15 minutes

Ingredients:

• 4 slices uncooked bacon

• 8 ounces ground beef (80% lean)

• 1 medium yellow onion, chopped

• 1 clove garlic, minced

• 3 cups beef broth

• 2 tablespoons tomato paste

• 2 teaspoons Dijon mustard

• Salt and pepper

• 1 cup shredded lettuce

• ½ cup shredded cheddar cheese

Instructions:

• Cook the bacon in a saucepan until crisp then drain on paper towels and chop.

• Reheat the bacon fat in the saucepan and add the beef.

• Cook until the beef is browned, then drain away half the fat.

• Reheat the saucepan and add the onion and garlic – cook for 6 minutes.

• Stir in the broth, tomato paste, and mustard then season with salt and pepper.

• Add the beef and simmer on medium-low for 15 minutes, covered.

• Spoon into bowls and top with shredded lettuce, cheddar cheese and bacon.

Nutrition Info: 315 calories, 20g fat, 27g protein, 6g carbs, 1g fiber, 5g net carbs

Grilled Pesto Salmon With Asparagus

• Servings: 4

• Prep Time: 5 minutes

• Cook Time: 15 minutes

Ingredients:

• 4 (6-ounce) boneless salmon fillets

• Salt and pepper

• 1 bunch asparagus, ends trimmed

• 2 tablespoons olive oil

• ¼ cup basil pesto

Instructions:

• Preheat a grill to high heat and oil the grates.

• Season the salmon with salt and pepper, then spray with cooking spray.

• Grill the salmon for 4 to 5 minutes on each side until cooked through.

• Toss the asparagus with oil and grill until tender, about 10 minutes.

• Spoon the pesto over the salmon and serve with the asparagus.

Nutrition Info: 300 calories, 17.5g fat, 34.5g protein, 2.5g carbs, 1.5g fiber, 1g net carbs